Clean Eating 101

How to Live a Healthy Lifestyle and Feel Better Everyday

By: Windy Madison

9781681279589

Publishers Notes

Disclaimer – Speedy Publishing LLC

This publication is intended to provide helpful and informative material. It is not intended to diagnose, treat, cure, or prevent any health problem or condition, nor is intended to replace the advice of a physician. No action should be taken solely on the contents of this book. Always consult your physician or qualified health-care professional on any matters regarding your health and before adopting any suggestions in this book or drawing inferences from it.

The author and publisher specifically disclaim all responsibility for any liability, loss or risk, personal or otherwise, which is incurred as a consequence, directly or indirectly, from the use or application of any contents of this book.

Any and all product names referenced within this book are the trademarks of their respective owners. None of these owners have sponsored, authorized, endorsed, or approved this book.

Always read all information provided by the manufacturers' product labels before using their products. The author and publisher are not responsible for claims made by manufacturers.

This book was originally printed before 2015. This is an adapted reprint by Speedy Publishing LLC with newly updated content designed to help readers with much more accurate and timely information and data.

Speedy Publishing LLC

40 E Main Street, Newark, Delaware, 19711

Contact Us: 1-888-248-4521

Website: http://www.speedypublishing.co

REPRINTED Paperback Edition: 9781681279589

Manufactured in the United States of America

Dedication

My beloved sister Lucy,

Being fit and living in a healthy lifestyle is very important.
You're my inspiration.

Table of Contents

Chapter 1- Understanding Clean Eating

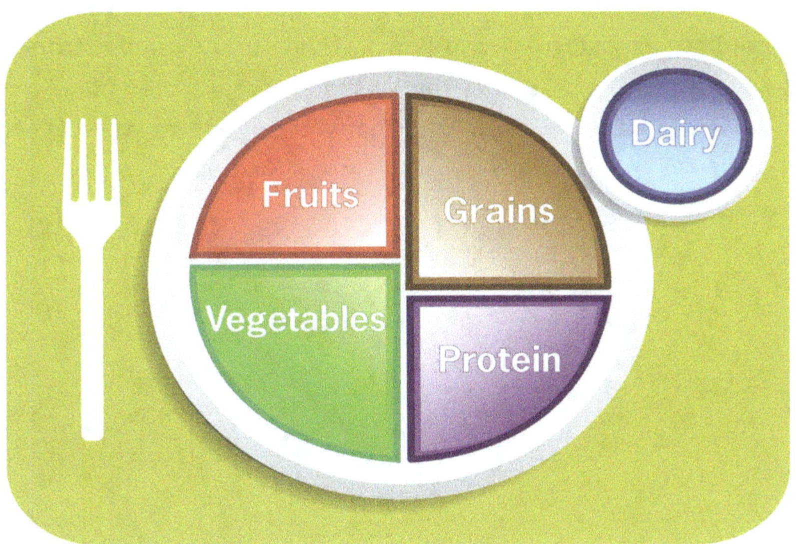

Most people know they need to improve their diets in one way or another. They also recognize how difficult this is when you drive down the street and you see a McDonald's on every corner or a line of fast food restaurants. Our lives have all become about convenience and in exchange for convenience we have become the most obese country in the world. With our instant gratification lifestyles we also know that eating healthy can be a challenge. However, it doesn't have to be this way and there are steps that you can take to balance out your life so that you can enjoy a Happy Meal with the kids on occasions.

Making your everyday diet healthier will allow you to improve the way you look, as well as the way you think. It's never too late to change your eating habits; you just have the personal motivation to do it.

Many people get stuck in ruts where they eat too much of one type of food. This leaves their body with excessive nutrients in one area, and none in another. No one likes to eat the same thing every day, but sometimes we do for the pure convenience of it.

There are a variety of foods that you can add to your diet to keep it from becoming stagnant and boring. There are hundreds of fruits and vegetables available at the average grocery store. There are also several other types of food that you can add to your CLEAN EATING DIET.

1. Fresh fruit

2. Vegetables

3. Meats

4. Whole grains

Variety is one of the things that nutritionists stress the most. They say that variety is important for both nutrition and psychological reasons. A varied diet is essential for a person to maintain good health and to maintain a good psychological well-being. Feeling deprived of your favorite foods can cause you to give up a healthy lifestyle. Variety allows you to incorporate your favorites with healthy foods and offers the chance for you to develop new favorites as well

It is important that you continue to eat foods that you like, but in moderation. Instead of giving up bacon, have it as occasional treat. The same is true for desserts and sweets.

Choosing healthy means that you want to look for foods that are not supped up with excess fat or sugar. It also means choosing meats from the lean section and removing the fat and skin from chicken. By doing this, you are eliminating unnecessary calories and excess fat.

When you choose breads and cereals, it is important not to choose those that are loaded with sugar or overly refined. Choose whole grains that have not been enhanced. Many of these whole grains are also fortified with additional vitamins and minerals. This insures that you are receiving these extra nutrients, but you should not rely on fortified foods alone. It is important that you get these nutrients in their natural form as well. Many foods are also supplemented with calcium and folic acid. These help to ensure that bones and teeth stay strong. Folic acid is essential in preventing birth defects.

If you can substitute healthy food for those that are less healthy, you will be on your way. For example, you can substitute skinless white meat chicken for dark meat drumsticks. This is a good way to maximize nutrition without losing good food options.

It is important that you choose a combination of foods that provide you with optimum nutrition. This means combining foods such as meats, beans, dairy and vegetables and whole grains to form a well-rounded meal. All of these foods combined together will provide you with the different nutrients that your body needs.

Most foods are obviously healthy. However, it may be difficult to know whether some items are healthy or not. In this instance, you will want to look at the nutritional labels. Labels are required on all packaged foods and can be very helpful to those who are looking to eat a healthier diet. Not only do the labels tell you how many calories, fat grams and other nutritional information, but they also provide detailed information on the type of vitamins and mineral are in the food as well.

When choosing healthy food, small changes can make a big difference. When you exchange fresh and low fat meals for high fat meals you will feel more energetic because you are not being "weighed down" by the high fat you were consuming in the past.

You feel full without feeling bloated. You should also notice an increase in energy levels.

By replacing highly processed grains for nutritious whole grains you will find that you are consuming more nutrients. Many of your highly refined foods are stripped of the nutrients and they do you little good in terms of a healthy diet.

By replacing highly processed grains for nutritious whole grains you will find that you are consuming more nutrients. Many of your highly refined foods are stripped on the nutrients and they do you little good in terms of a healthy diet.

Cooking techniques are also important. It is imperative that you don't cook with high fat oil, but use a cooking spread instead. This ensures that you are not eating any unnecessary fats in the form of oil. If you cook vegetables too long, you may actually be cooking away significant amounts of nutrients. Take broccoli as an example. If you over boil it and then slather it in butter and cheese, you are cooking away nutrients and replacing them with fat. Boiling it too long can also cause them to lose nutrients. To prepare vegetables, you are often better off quickly steaming them in the microwave or over the stove. Cook them in as little water as possible, but use enough to keep them from becoming scorched.

When you cook potatoes, it is good idea to include the skin. The skin contains a lot of fiber, nutrients and minerals. You can also cook a baked potato in the microwave or grill to give it a better flavor. By using these methods, you make the skin soft and minimized the need to load it with butter, sour cream, cheese, bacon, etc. In fact, healthier alternatives would include a little bit of nonfat cottage cheese or nonfat yogurt.

CHAPTER 2- WHAT ARE THE BENEFITS OF CLEAN EATING

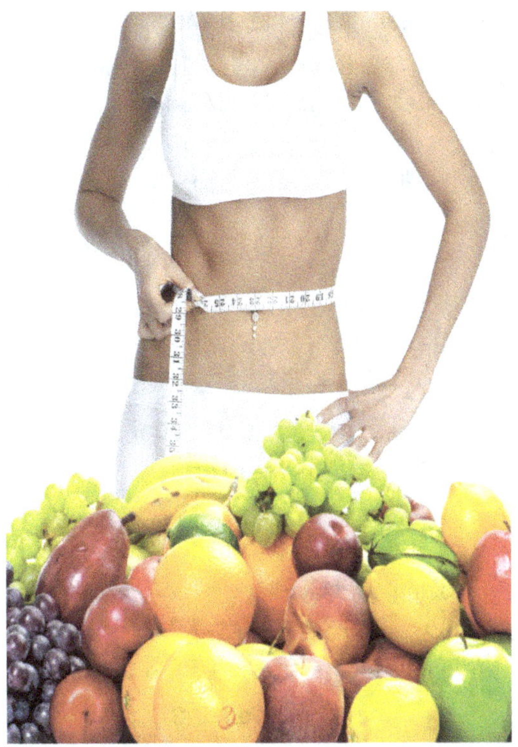

When it comes to eating, how many of us really bother to check whether we are having healthy food. Today's lifestyle has become so busy and hectic that you grab foods that taste good and tend to neglect its ill effect. There are several reasons and benefits of clean eating and thus you should remove time to prepare healthy food and chalk out a diet for a healthy living.

Here are the benefits of clean eating:

• The most important advantage is that you gain command over your weight. By eating correctly, you likewise make certain that your metabolic functions - most notably your immune system and your gastrointestinal system - keep working correctly. You're likewise protected from assorted chronic diseases, right from cardiovascular diseases like coronary artery disease and high blood pressure to diabetes.

● Eating healthy means you spend much less. Your bills at the supermarkets come down drastically and you don't plunge farther into charge card debt if that is already an issue with you. In addition to that, you save a huge bundle on all the healthcare expenses you'd need if any issue surfaces because of your food binging habits.

● A lot of foods nowadays are toxic because of the synthetic chemicals present in them. When you're attempting to eat correctly, you are much less likely to get these toxins into your body as one of the basic dogmas of eating correctly is that you shouldn't eat anything that's man-made.

In addition to that, if you eat less, you'll likewise be able to reduce on vices like smoking and alcoholism. A glass of beer is almost synonymous with a night out with the boys. If you eat less, you won't want the beer as well. Similarly, you will not want that one (or more) mandatory smoke that you tend to have after each meal.

● When you eat better, you'll find that you are able to do your work in a much better way. You are able to exercise more, travel more, play more, work more and therefore make your life more productive.

That sure beats being a fat slob and lounging around on the couch the whole day, doesn't it? You are able to also be more involved with your friends and loved ones and that surely enriches your life.

●Forget about fat fetishism, individuals who are overweight don't look appealing. There's a strong social taboo about weight on the wrong places of the body. If you're trying to find a partner, your flab may literally get in the way. Not simply that, individuals who can't control their eating habits and hence their weights are looked down upon by society as being individuals who can't control their basic urges.

This sort of psychology does exist, though very few individuals will speak about it. When you eat correctly, you'll discover that such issues disappear.

● Apart from feeling and looking good, your body will be high on energy, and fresh. With clean eating, you enjoy doing everything, and live a full life. Clean eating leads to a healthier you and you find little or no reason to visit a doctor. You can spend time in more activities to keep fit.

● As a healthy diet keeps the immune system stronger, and health problems are kept far away. A healthy immune system will take care that you stay fit and if sick to recover fast.

● Healthy diets help you stay in shape. A well-planned and healthy food helps to maintain your weight and you save yourself from the worry of losing or gaining weight.

● Your brain gets alert and sharp, which helps you to perform well in all your activities. A research has proved that a healthy diet helps your mind to think we'll even in the old age. You must have seen people fit and fine even in late 80's and all this is the result of proper food intake.

● A wholesome diet gives you all the essential minerals and nutrients that fulfill all the needs of your body.

● A healthy diet has proved to keep humans in a happy mood. Hence, you enjoy every moment of life and stay calm in every situation.

● Your skin is the face of your body. You know what the secret for a glowing skin is? It is healthy food. This not only makes you look great, but you feel strengthened from within.

● A good diet is very important for growing kids. Children are very active, burn lot of calories, and thus require all the required proteins, carbs, fats, and nutrients to stay fit and not affect their growth in any way.

Many people who have ignored bad eating habits have regretted in the older years. Healthy food keeps away many diseases and ill effects and you live a life that is free of tension and problems. Apart from enjoying life, you develop positive feelings.

Therefore, healthy food keeps both mind and body fit for life long. Thus, it is never too late to begin to eat healthy food and so live a healthy life. You will never run into bad effects because of good eating habits. So it is always better to eat well and stay in good shape. You can keep obesity and other harmful health problems far away from you.

CHAPTER 3- CLEAN EATING TO HAVE A HEALTHY LIFESTYLE

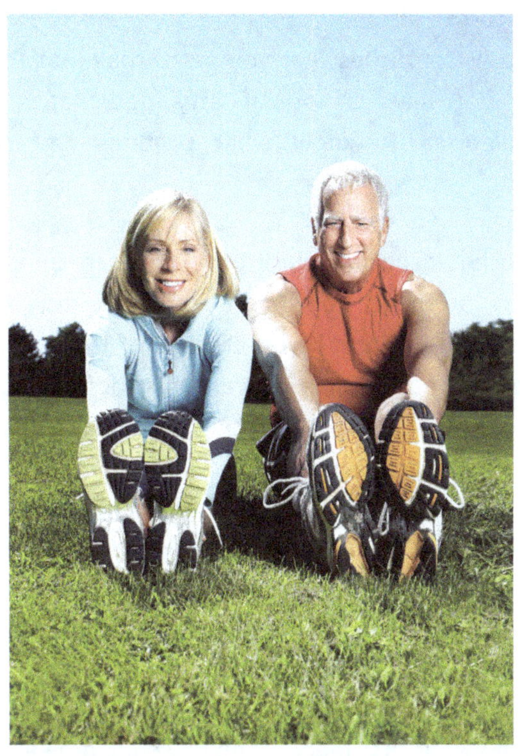

Clean Eating for Overweight

Seeing overweight persons has now become a common feature. Every other person is overweight, if not obese. Besides making a person look ungainly, obesity affects a person adversely, posing severe health hazards.

There are no advantages to being overweight, only disadvantages. If you are overweight and you want to lose that extra body fat, a perfect diet is essential. A diet that is chalked out considering your age, gender, and fat percentage and body weight would be a perfect diet.

Clean Eating 101

Visit a dietician, who is an expert in this field and share with him/her your eating habits and lifestyle. Here are a few tips on how you can start with a fat-loss program, which you could follow yourself.

Diet: Make a list of dishes that you eat throughout the day for a week. After that, make a note of fatty food that you consume. Consult a dietician to know what contains fat and what is nutritious.

Eliminate those items from your list that generate unnecessary fats in your body. If those items are your favorites, reduce their consumption to start with. If you are one of those, who overeat, then you need to have plenty of water just before you start your meal and if you feel hungry after every 2 hours, then try having salads or fruits, and not bananas.

There is nothing better than a fruit and vegetable diet. Some of the best foods are boiled vegetables, fruit salads, vegetable salads, etc., which supply vitamins and minerals for the body and make you fit.

Breakfast being your first meal of the day should be at about 7 am and must be heavy and nutritious. Lunch should be a little light at about 1 pm and your dinner has to be bare minimum by 7pm. Eating healthy meals on time is necessary for fat loss. Always follow the saying, "eat your breakfast alone, share your lunch with friends and give your dinner to your enemy".

Exercise: Exercise to lose extra body fats. Your work out should mainly consist of cardio vascular exercises, such as running, jogging, cycling, skipping, etc. Fat loss is the result of balanced combination of diet and exercise. Do not make the mistake of exercising vigorously, initially.

Many people get carried away with the whole weight loss spree and end up with severe body pain and miss out on further exercises. If you are used to exercising, you can very well go ahead with your work out and gradually increase exercising more.

Here is a tip on how to increase your metabolism rate and lose fats faster. Work out for the biggest muscle of your body, your legs. Consisting of quadriceps, hamstrings and calves, your legs have to be strong and not fat, as they carry your entire weight.

Other things: Reduce alcohol, aerated drinks, sweets, chocolates, oily foods, and other fattening edibles drastically. They contribute a lot to obesity. Overeating and continuous eating also adds to obesity. Obesity is one of the causes for cardiac arrests in many people. Therefore eat healthy, exercise well and beat obesity.

Clean Eating for Weight Gain

A lot is written about weight loss and a slimmer body. However, some are underweight, and constantly look for ways to gain weight. To stay healthy, one needs the perfect weight.

Being underweight is equally bad for your body. If you have tried to gain weight and failed every attempt, the reason may be that either you are following a wrong path or you are just not following the method.

Your body weight depends on what you eat. Eating unhealthy stuff can lead to weight loss and make you look pale and sick. When the body is deprived of proper meals, it will start eating the cells within the body making you lose your body mass.

Do you know that every time your body makes any movements, it loses calories? There are many people, who have a busy and hectic life, but simply fail to eat and neglect to eat what the body requires.

Eating healthy meals and at proper time will help you gain the perfect body shape that you have been wishing for. If you fall in the category of underweight persons, firstly, alter your diet and include foods that are more nutritious. Have small meals, but take it at least 4 to 5 times a day.

Apart from altering your diet, you need to change your eating habits as well. You can't keep eating as you wish. You should understand your body clock and work accordingly.

Long gaps between meals are as good as starving, and destroy your cells. Plan out a schedule to eat and follow it accordingly. Frequent changes affect the body adversely and make you lose more energy and body mass. Begin your day with a glass of milk and cereals, and then eat fruits.

Prepare a few vegetable sandwiches with butter or cheese. Remember to take your breakfast, soon after you wake up.

There should also be less time gap between your breakfast and lunch. If for any reason it takes time, grab a fruit or a healthy drink or a nutritious bar to munch. It is good to make salads as part of your meals.

A large portion of chicken or fish is healthy and helps you gain weight as well. It is a good idea to include some green leafy vegetables in your meals. Do take a snack break in the evening and pamper yourself with some protein drink and healthy sandwiches or salad.

If at any time you happen to do some heavy activities, remember your body has burnt lots of calories and thus you need to recharge by eating something healthy. Include a lot of liquids in your diet as well, so that the body keeps getting the required amount of liquid to flush out the unwanted toxins and keep your stomach clean.

Combining clean eating with exercise will do wonders for your body. A good diet will not only help you gain weight, but also make you look great. When your energy levels are high, you feel fresh throughout the day and can undertake any task with ease.

A healthy body and mind can do lots of good. Eat right and stay fit and you will enjoy life like never before. If you have a balanced diet, you need not consume weight gain powders or tablets. A proper diet should work perfectly on your body. Nothing is as great as eating good, wholesome food.

Clean Eating for Teenagers

Growing children need plenty of energy to perform their daily activities. An average teenager is involved in high intensity activities compared to an office worker. Activities can be low, medium, and high intensity. Study, play, exams, camps, trips, big games, tours, etc., are some of the many activities that form part of a teenager's life through the day. He/she needs both, mental and physical strength up with this routine, to remain fit and healthy.

A teenager's diet of should contain carbohydrates, proteins, minerals, vitamins, and all the essentials that their bodies need. A teenager should have more food as compared to a 45 year old. This is because teenagers have high metabolism rates. Five or six medium meals justify an average teenager's diet pattern.

A little bit of fatty food is again not a problem because the fats in the body disappear the moment they start engaging themselves in different games, trips or any other activities. In fact, teenagers should eat heavy meals, as this is their only time to build strong bodies.

The essential and healthy food items for a teenager are:

Milk - provides calcium for healthy teeth and bones. Water content n the milk keeps you hydrated.

Fruit juices - gives the teenager that little boost in stamina required while they play.

Water - an average teenager must consume at least 8-10 liters of water per day.

Meat and eggs - provides proteins, vitamins and carbohydrates. Very essential to increase weight and muscle mass. Fish helps in increasing concentration and alertness.

Fruits and vegetables - are more essential than non-vegetarian food. It is important because the minerals and vitamins are needed for the body and keeps the body hydrated. Fruits also help in learning and remembering. Dieticians recommend plenty of fruits and vegetables for growing teens. Fruits and vegetables are great to gain weight and remain fit.

All the above food items help teens in their studies and physical activities. The food cycle of an average teenager should be heavy breakfast at about seven, a fruit around 10, good lunch at about one, a fruit at about 3, and a small meal at around 5 with a fruit juice and dinner at 8.

A growing teen must not eat oily or fattening foods, as this might make him/her lazy, lethargic or even build excess body fats, which are the initial stages of obesity. If your teenager is not engaged in sports or exercises, absolutely do not follow the abovementioned foods, since with clean eating; there should always be good exercise.

Teens with low metabolism rate often put on more weight, even if they eat less. This is not correct. The idea is to eat healthy and exercise more to increase the metabolism rate and reduce the unwanted fats in the body.

Teens that are always attached to the computer or are at home should reduce the intake of meat, energy drinks, and milk, as it is not necessary for them and they might put on fats in their bodies. To conclude, teens should stop eating junk food from outside and stick to home cooked food to stay healthy and fit.

Clean Eating for People Over Sixty

Generally, people in over sixty have altered food tastes. Foods do not taste the same. They lose appetite and even their favorite foods do not fascinate them anymore. They tend to put on weight even if they barely eat.

Metabolism rates decrease with age and people tend to put on fats. Increasing weight in sixties is a bad sign, as it can cause many health related hazards. A person in his/her sixties must follow a proper diet plan. Here are some tips on how you can maintain your weight and diet accordingly.

People usually do not work very hard in their sixties and therefore need less energy, but just enough to perform daily chores. Your diet must contain adequate amount of protein, calcium, carbohydrates and vitamins.

Eat different varieties of food every day, so that it does not get monotonous and you have different taste every day. As you grow old, your bones tend to become weak and feeble. Your calcium level decreases and you are likely to suffer from osteoporosis.

To avoid these sufferings, you should drink enough low-fat milk and eat fat free dairy products like cheese and butter. Make sure you do not gain fat.

Fruits and vegetables are a very important source of nutrition for persons of this age group, as they provide a sufficient amount of vitamins and minerals. Most fruits contain vitamins B and C. Vitamins and calcium prevent memory loss, and shivering. Protein in your diet must only be about 15-18%, and mostly got from non-vegetarian foods like fish, eggs, and meat.

Always keep your body hydrated with water and juices. Water helps in cleansing the body from its impurities. Eat fiber rich food like vegetables that provide proteins, too. More of fiber in the body means less of toxins. Fiber can be found in pulses and baked beans, prunes and apricots.

Do not eat a lot of sweet or sugar based food because the empty calories present in them do not exactly provide energy, but increases weight. Consumption of excess salt may raise high blood pressure, therefore, control intakes of salt and sugar.

Since senior people do not exactly engage themselves in physical activity, regular exercise and a proper diet is a must. One has to increase metabolism rate, in order to remain fit and not put on excess weight. Old people often eat very less and cannot have three big meals. They must have small meals after regular intervals, which helps to increase their metabolism rate.

Do not take any protein supplements or fats loss pills because they need vigorous workouts and are basically meant for people below

Avoid canned or packed food items, as they contain preservatives, which are not healthy for persons of that age group.

Some packaged food also contains hydrogenated fats that may cause a problem in your cardio-vascular system. Eat controlled amounts of food, but ensure they are nutrient rich, so that you live a long, healthy life.

Clean Eating for Infants

As a parent, you must take a number of precautions about your infant's diet. The best food for an infant is mother's milk. Normally, an infant is considered as baby of age 0 – 1 year old.

People even consider preschoolers as infants. Let us categorize infants in different age groups and discuss their diet and precautions taken.

0-4 months: From the day of birth until the infant is 4 months, there is no better food for the child than the mother's milk. Mother's milk contains all the essentials that a child needs in balanced amounts. The temperature, thinness of milk, germ fighting and immunity enhancers, and many other factors ideal for the infant are present in mother's milk.

At this time, an infant is not ready to digest solid or semi-solid foods; therefore, continue breast-feeding until 4-5 months. Even if the baby gets diarrhea, continue breast-feeding. It is best to continue breast-feeding the child up to the age of one year, but in this age, it is not possible.

5-6 months: You can now introduce your child to semi-solid food. At this age, the baby is not completely ready to ingest semi-solid food, but is partially all right. Try to feed the baby with cereals like wheat, maize or mashed fruits like apples.

Make sure you dilute the food with either mother's milk or water. Feed the infant porridges. Feed the infant small amounts to a time, until it no longer is hungry.

Do not force-feed your infant, as it might initially not eat and might throw up. This happens because the infant is used only to sucking. The infant's food intake will gradually increase. Do not stop breast-feeding.

When your infant opens his/her mouth while feeding or the eyes follow the spoon means, your baby is now ready to taste and eat new food. Always feed your baby on your lap, this gives them the feeling of security.

7-9 months: After the baby gives positive response to the semi-solid food, you can now bring in mild solid food. Extremely small and fine pieces of fruits and vegetables, soft cheese, thin pieces of chicken should be the child's meal. Initially the child might not be very happy biting the food and might not eat.

Therefore it is advised not to stop breast-feeding. If your baby is hungry every 2-4 hours and wets the diapers 4-6 times a day, it means, your baby is getting food and fluids in right quantity. Other indication could be baby's weight increase.

10-12 months: The food in this period is not so different, but a little variation in the food is required. Bigger chopped piece of meat, fish, vegetables and fruits could be given. Cereals, mother's milk and fruit juices diluted with water are recommended as liquids. Always introduce new foods after every 2 weeks.

This helps you spot the food types that cause allergies or illness to your child. Maintain a high level of hygiene. Always boil water; always feed lukewarm food.

Chapter 4- Clean Eating on a Budget

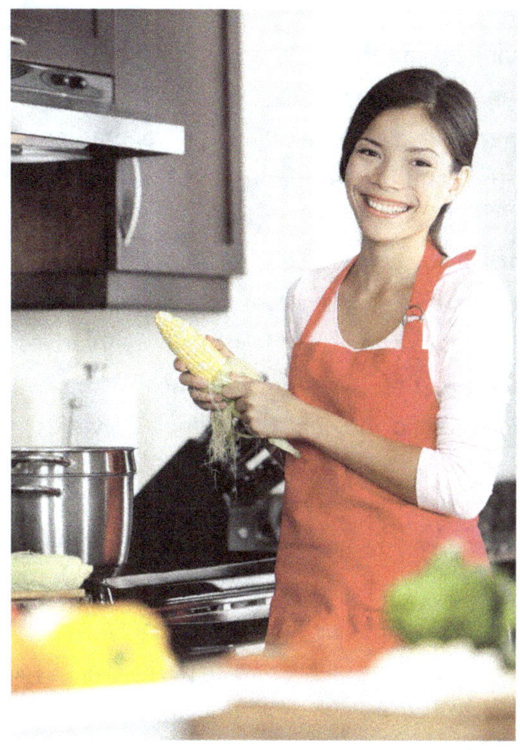

With food and fuel prices going through the roof, the world over, it has become very important to restrict even necessary expenses, and go on a budget. While it is essential to remain healthy, you can remain healthy on a budget. It is not difficult, when you know how. First, calculate the average monthly food expenses.

Include everything from day-to-day expenses for vegetables, fruits, meat and dairy products, and the money spent on going to restaurants and pubs, etc. Once you have the average figure of the past few months, it becomes a bit easier to plan your monthly budget. Since health is a priority, eliminate all the trips made to the local donut shop. You can still visit the donut shop, but restrict it to twice or three times a month. Substitute your donut break with fresh fruits or fruit or vegetable juices. If you need to eat something crunchy, then eat a whole-wheat cracker or a couple of biscuits with a vegetable salad, and the health benefits show up almost immediately.

The main savings come during your trip to the supermarket. Check local newspapers or magazines for special offers and use food coupons, wherever possible. Buy your vegetables and fruits in larger quantities, and if possible in bags, instead of buying it on a per-piece basis. It works out to be cheaper. Trimmed and cut vegetables are also costlier, so avoid buying them. Most of the supermarkets have special schemes for juices and other canned items. Buy the ones that do not have preservatives or artificial colors and stick to the 100% natural ones instead. While buying meat products, avoid buying the boneless variety, since it is costlier.

You can also remove the fat yourself from beef, instead of buying the costlier low fat variety. Avoid red meat as much as possible and stick to white meat like chicken. It is light on your wallet and your heart too. Eat more vegetables with pasta, spaghetti, rice, etc., instead of eating too much meat. Include potato, onions, garlic, ginger, and mint in your diet. These are not only comparatively cheap, but also strengthen your immune system. When cooked with vegetables, they convert the dish into a tasty masterpiece.

Change your breakfast menu, and in case you eat high fat and high calorie items, such as fried bacon, eggs, and white bread smothered in butter. Replace these items with oatmeal, whole meal bread, egg whites, and whole-wheat muffins. You can also make a smoothie by mixing bananas or strawberries in cold milk. It is inexpensive, yet filling. In case you want to eat bacon and egg, restrict yourself to eating it once or twice a week and grill it instead of frying it. Your dinner should also be light, yet filling. Try to make pizzas and burgers at home. They will turn out to be healthier and much cheaper compared to restaurants. Instead of visiting pubs regularly, call a few friends over and enjoy your drinks with wholesome homemade food.

So, instead of just complaining about high fuel and food prices over which you have no control, use it as an excuse to change to healthier eating habits. Combine clean eating with an exercise regimen to save money and to lead a long and healthy life.

Is the food you eat healthy? Does it contain all the proteins, minerals and vitamins essentials? If you don't already know, it's high time you realize what exactly you are consuming. The three meals of the day have to be healthy and on time; if possible stretch them to five or six smaller meals. If you are a working in an office or are a salesperson, you will tend to order some fast food, as and when you are hungry.

This is a very unhealthy idea. Make an effort, and cook something healthy. If you don't know how to cook or have any recipes, you can always search online. Many sites give you detailed recipes for vegetarian and non-vegetarian cooking.

Salads with fruits and vegetables are a very healthy meal for all ages. It provides you with a lot of energy and keeps you fit. A lot of doctors and dieticians recommend salad meal at least once in a day. If you get bored eating the same salad every day, add new flavors, and bring in a greater variety and try different methods of preparing salads. Grilled, baked, and steamed food is always advisable.

Many people do not eat healthy because most of them cannot give up the foods they like, which is fattening, but tasty. You can always add non-vegetarian items like boiled chicken, grilled pieces of steak, egg white and grilled bacon. This is mainly for people, who do not want to give up on steak and bacon easily. You can always search online for healthy recipes of foods that contain your favorite steak, bacon, ham, etc. Avoid eating fat content foods like egg yolk, bread, rice, sugar and sweets. Try brown and whole wheat bread and brown rice and brown sugar instead. There is always a healthy alternative for your taste of food. In your recipes, always use ingredients that are sugar free, cholesterol free and fat free. This helps you remain fit and reduces risks to your cardio vascular system.

Simple Facts:

- Avoid using too much oil

- Do not overeat

- Use right ingredients

- White, and lean meats are better than fatty red meat

- Dairy based products are fattening

- Avoid deep fried foods

- Processed food is not all that great, though it might taste good

- Junk food is filling but not healthy.

- Olive oil is the best cooking medium, if at all you want to deep-fry something.

- Instead of frying, stir-fry your vegetables.

Find time to search for food facts, what alternatives you can have etc. Learn ways to make meals with less fattening and yet healthy and tasty. Remember it's not only for you, but your family as well.

Windy Madison

Your recipe should never contain a lot of non-vegetarian food, especially if you are serving dinner because non-vegetarian food takes a bit longer to digest. Fruits and vegetables in all your food are healthy. If you have decided to cook and eat healthy food, check the difference in your weight, skin, freshness and concentration just in a few weeks.

Chapter 5- 101 Tips For Losing Weight Using Clean Eating

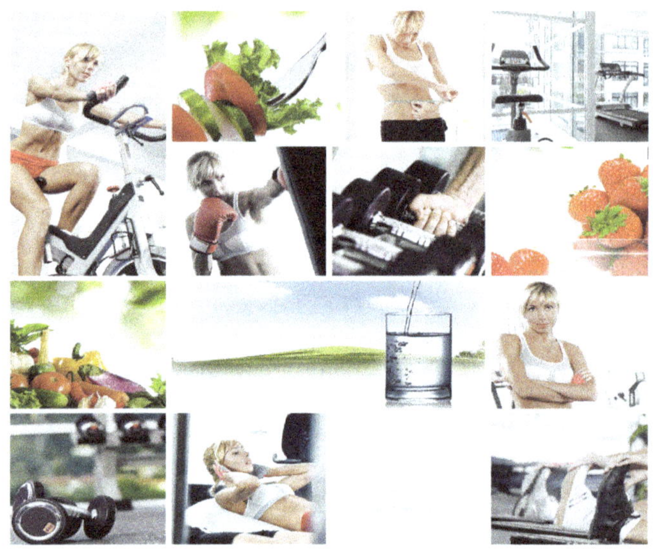

1. Drink plenty of water. Our body needs a lot of water so give in to water. Water is not just way to flush out toxin but if you have more water in your body you will generally feel healthier and fitter. The best thing about water is that is has no calories at all.

2. Start your day with a glass of water. As soon as you wake up, gulp down a glass of cool water. It's a wonderful way to start you day and you only need a lesser quantity of your breakfast drink after that. A glass of water lets out all your digestive juices and sort of lubricates the insides of your body. You may have your morning cup of tea but have it after a glass of water. It is good for you.

3. Drink a glass of water before you start the meal. Water naturally needs some space so that you feel fuller without actually having to stuff yourself.

4. Have another glass of water while you are having the meal. Again this is another way of making yourself full so that you can actually rise from the table eating less but feeling full just the same. Instead of drinking it one gulp, take sips after each morsel. It will

help the food to settle faster so that you get that feeling that you are full faster.

SIDENOTE: Water is such a remarkable thing, but seldom do we give it the credit that it deserves. Did you know that over 66% of your body weight is nothing but water? It's amazing!

5. Stay away from sweetened bottle drinks, especially sodas. Hey all those colas and fizzy drinks are sweetened with sugar and sugar means calories. The more you can cut out on these sweetened bottle drinks, the better for you. So if you must drink sodas, then stick to diet sodas.

6. Include in your diet things that contain more water like tomatoes and watermelons. These things contain 90 to 95 % water so that there is nothing that you have to lose by feasting on them. They fill you up without adding to the pounds.

7. Eat fresh fruit instead of drinking fruit juice. Juice is often sweetened but fresh fruits have natural sugars. When you eat fruit, you are taking in a lot of fiber, which is needed by the body, and fruits of course are an excellent source of vitamins.

8. If you do have a craving for fruit juice then go for fresh fruit juice instead of these that contain artificial flavors and colors. Or even better, try making your own fruit juice taking care not to sweeten it with too many calories.

9. Choose fresh fruit to processed fruits. Processed and canned fruits do not have as much fiber as fresh fruit and processed and canned fruits are nearly always sweetened.

10. Increase your fiber intake. Like I mentioned, the body needs a lot of fiber. So try to include in your diet as many fruits and vegetables as you can.

11. Go crazy on vegetables. Vegetables are your best bet when it comes to losing pounds. Nature has a terrific spread when it comes to choosing vegetables. And the leafy green vegetables are your best bet. Try to include a salad in your diet always.

12. Eat intelligently. The difference between man and beast is that we are driven by intelligence while beasts are driven by instinct. Don't just eat something because you feel like eating it. Ask yourself whether your body really needs it.

13. Watch what you eat. Keep a watchful eye on everything that goes in. Sometimes the garnishes can richer than the food itself. Accompaniments too can be very rich. Remember that it is the easiest thing in the world to eat something without realizing that it was something that you should not have eaten.

14. Control that sweet tooth. Remember that sweet things generally mean more calories. It is natural that we have cravings for sweet things especially chocolates and other confectionary. Go easy on these things and each time you consume something sweet understand that it is going to add on somewhere.

15. Fix times to have meals and stick to it. Try to have food at fixed times of the day. You can stretch these times by half an hour, but anything more than that is going to affect your eating pattern, the result will either be a loss of appetite or that famished feeling which will make you stuff yourself with more than what is required the next time you eat.

16. Eat only when you are hungry. Some of us have the tendency to eat whenever we see food. We use parties as an excuse to stuff our selves. Understand that the effect of a whole week of dieting can be wasted by just one day's party food. Whenever you are offered something to eat do not decline it completely bit just break of a nibble so that you appear to mind your manners and at the same time can watch your diet.

17. Quit snacking in between meals. Do not fall for snacks in between meals. This is especially true for those who have to travel a lot. They feel that the only time they can get a bite to eat is snacks and junk food. The main problem with most snacks and junk food is that they are usually less filling and contain a lot of fat and calories. Just think about French fries…tempting but terribly fattening.

18. Snack on vegetables if you must. You might get the pangs of hunger in between meals. It is something that you can very well control or even better, try munching on carrots. They are an excellent way to satisfy those hungry pangs and are good for your eyes and teeth. True, you might end up being called Bugs Bunny, but its miles better to be called Bugs Bunny than fatso.

19. Go easy on tea and coffee. Tea and coffee are harmless by themselves. It's when you add the cream and sugar that they become fattening. Did you know that having a cup of tea or coffee that has cream and at least two cubes of sugar is as bad as having a big piece of rich chocolate cake?

20. Try to stick to black tea/coffee. Black tea or coffee can actually be good for you. But personally I would like to recommend tea rather than coffee. The caffeine in the coffee is not really good for you because it is an alkaloid and can affect other functions of your body like the metabolism.

21. Count the calories as you eat. It's a good idea to have an idea of the calories that most food items have. If it is a packed thing then the label is sure to have the calories that the substance has.

22. Be sure to burn out those extra calories by the end of the week. If you feel that you have consumed more calories than you should have during the week, it happens you know, and then make sure that you work off those extra calories by the end of the week.

23. Stay away from fried things. Fried things are an absolute no-no. The more fried things that you avoid, the lesser weight you will gain. Fried things are called so because they are fried in oil or fat. And even if the external oil is drained away, there is still a lot of hidden oil in it so stay away from it.

24. Do not skip meals. The worst thing you can do while watching you diet is skip a meal. It has just the opposite effect of what you want. You need to have at least four regular meals every day.

25. Fresh vegetables are better than cooked or canned vegetables. Try to eat your vegetables raw. When you cook them, you are in fact taking away nearly half the vitamins in them. And canned vegetables too are processed and are not nearly half as good as fresh vegetables. When you buy your vegetables it would be a good thing to see if the label says that it is pesticide free.

26. Nothing more than an egg a day. Eggs are not such a bright idea. It would be best to reduce your intake of eggs to maybe three in a week. But for those of you die hard egg fans, you may have up to one egg a day but nothing more than that.

27. Make chocolates a luxury and not a routine. Chocolates are not or at least they should not be a part of your diet. So do not indulge too much in them. Even the bitter chocolates are not good for you because though the sugar is less there is still the cream in them.

28. Choose a variety of foods from all food groups every day. This is a fine way of keeping deficiency diseases at bay. Change the items included in your diet every day. This is an excellent way of keeping deficiency diseases at bay and it helps you to experiment with a variety of dishes and thereby you do not get bored of your diet.

29. If you can say no to alcoholic beverages please do. Alcoholic beverages too are not good for you. Beer can be fattening and the rest of the alcoholic drinks may not be fattening by themselves but

after a couple of swigs you will be in no position to watch your diet and your appetite too will be something to battle with.

30. Try to have breakfast within one hour of waking. It's always best to have breakfast within an hour of waking so that your body can charge itself with the energy it needs for the day. The idea is not to wait for you to get really hungry. Breakfast is the most important meal of the day but that does not mean that it should be the most filling meal of the day.

31. 50 to 55% of your diet should be carbohydrates. It is a myth that you should try and avoid carbohydrates when you are on a diet. Rather the other way round I should say. Carbohydrates are a ready source of energy and so 50 to 55% of your diet should be carbohydrates.

32. 25 to 30% of your diet should be proteins. Various processes and activities are going on in our bodies. Things are broken down and being built up again. Resistance has to be built up, recovery from disease too is needed and for all this the body needs plenty of proteins so see to it that 25 to 30 % of your diet consists of proteins.

33. Fats should only be 15 to 20 %. You need only this much of fat in your diet so keep it at that.

34. Try and adopt a vegetarian diet. A vegetarian diet is undoubtedly better for those of us watching our diet. There are a lot of advantages of keeping to a vegetarian diet but I don't want to sing an ode to vegetarianism now. What I would suggest is keep to a vegetarian diet as much as you can. Make a non- vegetarian diet a week end event or something if you find it impossible to give up eating all those animals.

35. Choose white meat rather than red. White meat, which includes fish and fowl, is miles better than red meat, which includes beef and pork for those trying to lose weight.

36. High Fiber multigrain breads are better than white breads. Remember how I told you to increase the fiber content in your food; well this is the answer to that. It is not only better in terms of the fiber content but also in terms of the protein content as well.

37. Reduce your intake of pork. Pork is not something that can help you to lose weight. So the lesser pork you eat the better chances you have of losing weight. And remember that pork includes the pork products as well, things like bacon, ham and sausages.

38. Limit your sugar intake. If you can't have things unsweetened go for sugar substitutes. These things are just as sweetening but are certainly not fattening.

39. Graze 5 to 6 times a day. Instead of sticking to just three meals a day, try grazing. Grazing means try having 5 or 6 smaller meals instead of three king sized meals. It is an excellent way of having smaller quantities of food.

40. Go ahead eat cheat food, but only for flavor. There are many things which you have to avoid from your diet but which you may have an undying craving for. Do not avoid them altogether. You could call them cheat foods and indulge in them once in a while. But take care just to tingle your taste buds, don't hog on them. Instead of that share them with others. In this way

41. Watch your fat intake. Each fat gram contains 9 calories so by reading the total calories on a food and knowing the quantity of fat, you can estimate the % of fat, which should in no way exceed 30% of the food.

42. Go easy on salt, as too much salt is one of the causes of obesity. Make it a point to really cut down on salt. Try to bring down your salt intake to half of what it was last year.

43. Change from table butter to cholesterol free butter. If you have a choice why not g for it, any way it is healthier for you and tastes just the same. Bear in mind that these small changes can go a long way towards weight reduction.

44. Instead of frying things try baking them without fat. Baking is by far a healthier method of preparing food than frying. Baking requires lesser oil or fat.

45. Use a non stick frying pan for your cooking so that you do not have to add oil. The golden rule is to try and avoid as much oil as possible and a non stick pan is the perfect solution to this problem.

46. Boil your vegetables instead of cooking them, or even better, eat them fresh. However if you do not like eating your vegetables as it is, try steaming them without adding anything at all. This is probably the healthiest way to eat cabbages, cauliflowers and a host of other vegetables.

47. Carry parsley with you. Parsley is an excellent thing to munch on in between meals. Not just is it good for you in terms of vitamins, but it is also a perfect way of making your breath fresher.

48. Choose low fat substitutes or no fat substitutes. There are plenty of low fat or even no fat substitutes available in the market so why not choose wisely. It is much better for you heart too. Many people just go for shopping and pick up whatever they can. They do not bother to find out if there are nay substitutes for the thing they are looking for.

In the markets of today, you will be astounded at the range of goods that manufactures have to offer. In fact with all the hue and cry that is being made about weight loss, low fat substitutes and no fat substitutes are hitting the stands faster than mushrooms that sprout after the first rains.

So the next time you head for the stores instead of picking up what you have always picked up, see if there are better substitutes.

Remember that our bodies need nutrients and not just calories. Fats give us nutrients but with more calories than what proteins or carbohydrates do.

49. Avoid crash diets. They are bad for health and you will gain what you have lost once you take a break. Crash diets are not a solution to weight loss. It might seem as if you have lost few pounds but the moment you give up on the crash diet everything will bounce back with a vengeance.

Take a look at it in this way. Do you think that it is possible for a person to survive on a crash diet for the rest of his or her life? Certainly not! So at some time or the other, you will have to give up the crash diet and then you will see for yourself that a crash diet does more harm than good on the long run.

Crash diets may have a lot to promise, but very rarely do these promises ring true. Crash diets are things people go on in order to wear an old dress or suit for a particular occasion. That's the only purpose that they serve as far as I can see.

50. God gave us teeth for a reason. Therefore we should develop a habit of chewing all food including liquid food and soft foods like sweets, ice creams at least 8 to 12 times. This is essential to add saliva to the food, as it is only in the saliva that sugar is digested.

Often we find that whatever goes into our mouth goes down like lightning. We hardly give the saliva any time to act on the food. So does digestion take place like it should? Do we just stuff our tummies with food that doesn't get digested or in other words that doesn't yield the benefits that it should?

51. Dry wine is better than sweet wine. Sweet wines naturally contain a lot of sugar. But on the other hand, in dry wines most of this sugar has been fermented away so from the weight point of view dry wines are better than sweet wines.

52. When you decide it's time to start working out, start slowly and don't get discouraged if you don't achieve your fitness goals after the first week. Many people make this mistake. They feel that if they really push their bodies they can lose more weight in a couple of work outs. This is a very serious thing in fact.

If you try to push your body too much in the first few goes, you are likely to end up with sprained joints, a sore back and even torn ligaments. The rule to be followed here is slow and steady wins the race.

53. Check your weight before you start the routine and keep checking for changes but do not expect a radical change immediately, it might be one or two weeks before you notice some change. However it is crucial that you continue to monitor your weight. You may bear in mind the fact that even a few pounds loss is a big achievement.

54. When you do notice a change, reward yourself. When I say reward I do not mean go for some goodies like chocolates or sweets. Maybe you could go for a movie or buy yourself something like a new dress or a trinket.

This is something that can keep you going. It is a good idea to save on the money that you wanted to spend on ice creams and chocolates and then treat yourself to something more substantial.

55. You can take a day off from exercise every week. This is not just a very good idea but it is part of the exercise routine. Your body needs a day off from an exercise routine so do not hesitate to take a day off from whatever you have been doing.

56. Exercise outdoors as far as possible. There are two advantages of doing whatever you are doing outside. One advantage is that it gives your body a chance to get a lot of the much needed fresh air and sunshine.

The second advantage is that the surroundings keep you perked up and it is a break from remaining cooped up all day long

57. Try to collect some information about exercise, there are a lot of things that you can do at home. Extensive research has been done on exercise and plenty of this information is easily available.

You can try browsing the net or getting a book or two on how to exercise at home. This information will be useful to you to know how much you need to work out on each specific exercise in order to burn off the desired number of calories.

58. Try to get somebody to exercise along with you. But it should be somebody committed or else your interest might dwindle. This is indeed an excellent idea. One of the advantages of getting a committed person t exercise with you is that it keeps you going. There may be days when you feel just too lazy to crawl out of bed in the mornings. On such days, the knowledge that somebody is waiting for you is enough to slide out of bed.

Another advantage is that you can discuss your progress and fears with another person and be a sympathetic listener to the other person as well. This is a fine way of getting motivated yourself.

59. Stop when your body has had enough. There is no sense in pushing it. When you have worked out for a considerable time, your body will start giving you signals.

Heed those signals. This is particularly true in the initial stages. Take one step at a time. Stop when you are out of breath or when a certain part of your body tells you that it has had enough.

60. If you want to increase your time of exercise or your workout routine, do it gradually and not in sudden steps.

Well easier said than done. Most of us have such hectic schedules that it is quite impossible to fit in tie for exercise right? Your body or anybody's body for that matter needs proper exercise. If you make up your mind to do it, you just can.

61. Select an exercise pattern to suit your life style. All f us have different life styles and professions so there is no sense in trying to follow the book strictly. Try and follow an exercise routine that is suitable for you. You have to understand that it is even more important than the exercise itself.

62. Don't stand, walk. If you can walk about then do so. Do not stand in a fixed position. Pacing about is a good thing to do. If you are thinking deeply about something, try pacing about, it will aid in your thinking.

63. Don't sit, stand. If you can stand, then do not sit. The golden rule is to choose a position that is less comfortable.

64. Don't lie down, sit. The rule that we mentioned above rings true here as well.

65. Do not be a couch potato. It is the easiest thing in the world to become a couch potato. You know what we are talking about don't you? That shapeless thing that sits or reclines on a shapeless chair in front of the television and stupidly munches away at something fried!

If you are inclined to become a promising old couch potato, break the habit, cut at the very root of the vine. Take away that favorite chair of yours. In fact, it would be a very good idea if you could keep a chair that isn't too comfortable in front of the TV. This will discourage any tendency to become a couch potato.

66. If you have a sitting job, stand up and stretch yourself every half an hour. Most of the jobs today are indeed sitting jobs that are in one word sedentary. This is especially true for those who sit and punch away at the keyboard or toy with the mouse all day long.

So if you have such a job, make it a point to get up at least every half an hour and stretch yourself.

67.

While making telephone calls try walking up and down. I hope you will agree with me that this is an excellent suggestion.

68. Use the stairs instead of the elevator whenever you can. Elevators are one hell of a convenience particularly if you have to go up or down some twenty floors. But elevators also make us very lazy.

There may be no sense in trudging up some twenty flights of stairs because by the time you get there you will be totally pooped. But while coming down, if you have the time, you can easily come down the stairs instead of using the elevator. Coming down is not at all exhausting.

And talking about the time factor, I don't think that there is much of a difference. Sometimes waiting for an elevator door to open at your floor after you hit the button can take up all of eternity.

69. Smoking is bad for weight loss. Smoking as such may not contribute to weight loss but smoking leads to other conditions like erratic eating habits and excessive dependence on things like coffee.

70. If you hate running, remember, you do not have to run a marathon to stay fit. 10 minutes of cardio each day is good enough for most.

71. And if you can't run, try walking. 15 minutes of brisk walking a day is enough to keep most fit.

72. Consider walking to places that you would normally drive (such as work or the market if they're not too far away). It may take you longer, but the health benefits will last you a lifetime.

73. It sounds strange, but some people have reported that they lost more weight when they drank black coffee before a workout. While there's no hard data to support this, nutritionists speculate that the caffeine in coffee makes the body rely more on fat for fuel during the work out.

74. Here's a corollary to the tip above: Avoid drinking coffee in excess, as it tends to desensitize your body to the fat burning effects of caffeine.

75. Stop using remote controls. Remote controls are the bane of a prospective weight loser. They may be remarkable gadgets by themselves but from the weight loss point of view, they just aren't very helpful.

They really encourage us to take a laid back kind of attitude towards life itself. In fact if remote controls were not there, the television would not have become so popular. It is because of remote controls that people can remain where they are and switch from one channel to the other. And they only have to twitch a finger muscle to achieve this.

Now, I have nothing against multi channel television sets but what I strongly advocate is that you get up from where you are and change the channel of the TV each time you want to do so.

The same thing holds true for other remote controls as well. As it is we have remote controlled TVs, DVD players, A/Cs, garage doors, gateways and what not. The next thing we know is that we will have remote controlled people as well.

76. Doing things that you can do by yourself like fetching, turning things off and on. Often when we come back tired from work, we tend to get others to do simple chores for us. These things are no big deal. They are things that we can very well do for ourselves but we don't.

That is why we often ask our kids to fetch us this or take away that.

Training your pet is a wonderful thing indeed. It is quite remarkable how some people get their dogs to fetch them something. But the fact is that while you may be making sure that your dog is getting a lot of exercise, you are neglecting your bit of the story.

77. Here's a pop quiz. Escalators help us to:

> 1. Move up and down faster
>
> 2. Gain weight
>
> 3. Stand stupidly as they move up and down
>
> 4. Look down at other people when you are going down
>
> 5. Look up to others when we are going up

You have to pick the correct answer from the 5 alternatives given. You can see for yourself that all the options are in a way correct. So the next time you travel on an escalator, don't just stand there...climb up or down along with it. (Or better yet, take the stairs.)

78. During commercial breaks walk about. If you want to sit all evening with your eyes glued to the tube, then do so. But at least spare your eyes the agony of a commercial break.

When the next commercial flashes on screen, instead of surfing, get up and take a walk. Reach over and try to touch your toes or do any such simple exercise that will at least get the blood flowing in your veins.

79. Wriggle your toes and your fingers whenever you can. This too is a stress buster and it gives you a chance to at least work your hand and leg joints. This will tell you how sore they are and if their condition is so bad, just think of the rest of your body.

80. Turn on music and dance like wild. Let your hair down once in a while. Go back to the days of wild child hood. Close the door of your room, turn on your sound system to the highest volume possible (but a little lower than the level at which your neighbors start to complain) and then do the wackiest dance that you can think of. Jump on your bed and jump off it again.

Roll all over the floor. Pretend that you are Michael Jackson or Madonna (you will never see them keeping still) and do ever boogie move that you know.

81. Carry a soft flying disc or Frisbee with you. Toss it around and get up to fetch it. This is also an excellent way to beat stress. It makes a person feel good to throw something away forcefully when the person is all worked up. And the thing that you throw is something soft and can't damage anything, and then what is stopping you?

It is not really the throwing part that we are interested in. It is the fetching part. Each time you get up to fetch it back; you are giving yourself a chance to stretch those muscles and joints

82. Get down at a block before your destination and walk the rest of the way. You might not have time to fit in long walks in your busy schedule so this is one way of ensuring that you at least get to walk for a little bit every day. If you take the bus or the subway, get down at an earlier station and see if you can walk the rest of the way.

If you drive to work, see if you can get space in a parking lot that is a little away from your office.

83. When nobody is watching try doing pelvic gyrations. If you take a moment to observe it you will see that it is the mid section of our body that gets the least bit of exercise and that is probably why the signs of weight gain are mostly seen there.

It is the same reason why we find it very difficult to lose weight in that section. So the best thing that you can do is consciously try to give that part a little bit of exercise.

Stomach crunches might be too strenuous an exercise to start off with but gyrations are relatively mild. Pelvic gyrations make you thrust your midsection towards all directions and this is the best way of tightening every muscle in that mid section and that is of course what weight loss is all about.

84. Tuck in your tummy whenever you walk. Get that proper gait. And the best way for that is to tuck in your tummy and inflate your chest. Do not let your tummy hang above your belt line like some unruly layer of flesh. Bring it under the belt.

Each time you tuck in your tummy, you will feel the pressure on the muscles of your stomach. This tightening and loosening of these muscles is even better than stomach crunches.

85. Try breathing exercises. You might be surprised to know that breathing exercises too can lead to weight loss. If you are doing the breathing exercises properly, you will find that you can exert a lot of pressure on the muscles around the mid section.

You can feel a tightening of these muscles each time you breathe in or breathe out. So go ahead and breathe properly, it is good for you.

86. Try yoga. Yoga is one of the best ways of losing weight. Of course I can't go into a full lecture about yoga over here but I can tell you that I have never seen people with better-toned bodies than those who practice yoga.

One of the benefits of yoga is that you learn to control virtually every muscle and joint of your body so that the issue of weight gain will cease to exist.

87. Try massaging your partner. This is a fun way to lose weight. It is something that can give your partner a lot of pleasure and at the same time can give you a lot of exertion there by leading to weight loss.

The attitude over here should of course be you scratch my back I will scratch yours. It should not be a one sided effort or else the interest will soon dwindle.

In fact it is a good idea if couples take up weight loss routines together. They can keep watch over each other, help control those urges to eat and motivate each other to stick to the routine.

There are a lot of things that couples can do together that can help them to keep physically active.

88. If you can't think of anything else to do try punching your pillow. Now here's another one of those weird ideas but believe me it works. Not too many of us have punching bags at home and if you have really fluffy pillow giving it a good punching routine is just as good as anything else.

This is also a nice way of letting off steam so go for it. After all something is better than nothing. But I would suggest that you do not hit it too violently or else the stuffing might come out. Do not bother too much about the force with which you hit the pillow. It is number of hits that are important. Try to get at least fifty punches in one bout.

If there is somebody that you particularly dislike like your boss or your neighbor, or may be your ex boy friend or girl friend, try fixing a picture of the persons head on the top of your pillow and then try punching it. I promise you, it will give you a lot of satisfaction.

89. Instead of waddling up and down the staircase, try taking them two at a time. Now this is something that you have to be careful about because we do not want you to trip. So when you do this make sure that your feet are well and truly planted on each step before you increase the beat and try two at a time.

90. If you have a dog, take it for a run and let the dog lead you on. You will be surprised as to how much exercise a dog can give you.

Animals are sensible enough to know that they need a lot of exercise so let your animal lead you on. Take your pet dog out for as walk and before you know what hit you, it will turn out to be a run.

91. Join a dance class. Dancing is a wonderful way to burn off those extra calories. It is true. When you dance you are in fact burning away a lot of calories. Of course we are not referring to the slow ballroom kind of dances in which one person actually leans on the other one for support. We are talking about fast dances.

The best way to do it is by joining a dance class because they will really wok you out. But I would suggest that you wait for a couple more pounds to vanish before you think of becoming a ballerina.

92. Whenever you can, lean against a wall with your hands flattened against the wall and in such a way that your face is very close to the wall. Then use your hands to push your body away from the wall. Do these two or three times at a stretch.

93. If there is a pool nearby go for swims as often as you can, swimming is one of the best exercises. Water has a lot of

advantages. And if nothing else, a cool dip in a pool is a wonderful stress reliever.

94. Try playing something like table tennis or basket ball. Games are a fun way to lose weight. It is much more exciting to play a game than just work out by yourself. The best thing about games is that they are addictive. Once you start playing you will soon end up with a friends' circle and then the playing goes on without even you knowing it.

It is something that you can look forward to and there is no stress involved in this program. In fact the more you play the less you will consider this to be a part of your weight loss program. As you burn away those calories, you will also be able to expand your social circle.

95. Any work out should start with a 5 to 10 minute warm up and should end with a 5 to ten minute cool down session. Whatever physical exercise you are involved in, you must remember to warm up before the exercise really starts. Do not just plunge into the water and start thrashing about, to put it figuratively.

Your body needs to reach a certain level of readiness before it can actually start responding to exercise. And this readiness is achieved by the warming up process.

96. Do not carry your mobile phone around but leave it a place where you can hear it ringing. In this way you make sure that you at least get up and walk towards it. This might sound sill but I really mean it. You need a reason to keep yourself going.

Life today has become so easy that we have everything at our fingertips. All we have to do is push a button here and push a button there. The only things that get any exercise at all are our fingers. Years ago Charles Darwin put forward a theory of use and disuse.

According to this theory, a certain part of the body that is put to constant use develops a lot and a certain part of the body that has no use at all becomes smaller and smaller and gradually ceases to exist.

Here are a certain examples that he quoted, were the long neck of the giraffe, which appeared to become longer and longer when the giraffe stretched higher and higher to reach the leaves at the treetops. He quoted the example of the absence of a tail in human beings to illustrate the example of the theory of disuse.

Now if Darwin's theory were to prove true, as the years go by man is likely to end up with just a huge head, a few fingers and maybe some other parts of the bodies that are also put to use.

That is why I made it a point to say that you have to drive yourself to move about. A cell phone may be convenient, but the same thing can turn out to simplify life just a little too bit. There are other arguments against the use of cell phones but that is beside our topic.

What I would suggest is that at home or in your office, leave the cell phone lying about so that you can hear it ring, but can't just reach into your pocket and answer it. See to it that you have to actually stand up and walk a few steps before you can pick it up.

97. While traveling in an elevator instead of just standing there and staring stupidly at the numbers going up or down, try raising yourself onto your toes and then back on your feet again. Do this several times. Also try flexing your buttock muscles as well.

In fact there are many muscles in our body that we can twitch and flex without inviting the attention of others. Even if others do notice you, it's no big deal provided you are flexing a muscle in a decent part of the body. (Most of the other parts do not have muscles any way.) Others might brand you as a health freak but it is miles better to be known as a heath freak than as a sack of potatoes.

98. Undress and stare at yourself in front of your mirror. If what you see displeases you, then you have all the more reason to work out. Try tucking in the extra fat in all those wide areas, this will give you an idea of which part you need to be working on.

Turn to you side and get a very good view of your side profile. This is an excellent way of checking whether you have a tummy that is starting to bulge or has bulged already.

Try pulling in air and then take a look at your tummy; if it has gone in even a little bit, there is hope for you. If you start now, you can control it where it is now and may be if you really set your mind to it; you can lose a couple of inches in a just a few weeks.

Weighing yourself on your bathroom scales is a good idea but viewing yourself in the. To be very frank, a few pounds gain may shock you but does not really disgust you. But a flabby figure and extra fat certainly will.

99. If you have a banister rail or a balustrade that will support you, sit on it and pump your legs as if you are riding a bicycle, taking care not to fall off of course. This might sound like another crazy idea. It is a way of keeping your mind alert all the time. Everything must look like an opportunity to you.

100. Do not slouch in your chair but try to maintain an erect posture with your tummy tucked in. Slouching is a very bad habit. Not only is it bad for your back but it also gives you a very flabby figure. It is your way of saying yes to a comfortable, weight-gaining pose.

Make it a point to always sit as erect as you can. It is also a terrific way to ward off back problems.

101. Most of us tend to put on weight particularly in the mid section. It is the tummy that seems to have a mind of its own. Mind you this doesn't hold true for post pregnancy tummies. This is what you have to do.

Breathe in air as strongly as you can and as you do so, tuck in your tummy as much as you can. Hold it like this for a few seconds and then slowly release your breath taking care not to let out your tummy. Try to keep breathing like this at least fifty or sixty times in a day.

In fact breathe like this whenever you can remember to do so. After the first day, you should feel the muscles of your stomach tightening each time you do this. Then you know that you are on the right track. If you practice this without fail for 20 days, at the end of the twentieth day, you will have lost at least an inch.

Below I have included a table of the various exercises and the number of calories that can be burnt with each exercise. Choose what you can do best and choose something that you will enjoy doing on the long run as well.

The choice of the exercise is completely left to you but try to do whatever you wish to do for at least twenty minutes. It is only after you do the exercise for twenty minutes that the actual calorie burning sets in.

Aerobics	200-250 calories
Bicycling, Stationary	250-300 calories
Bicycling, Actual	300-400 calories

Running, 5-6 mph	300-350 calories
Stair climber	200-250 calories
Swimming laps	350 calories
Walking briskly	150-180 calories

From this you can see for yourself that walking is not at all something that has to be sidelined. If you really find your days to be too full to fit in any other form of exercise, then walking is your best bet. Walk as much as you can.

Try getting to places and leaving places a little early. This will give you time to walk.

The ball is now in your court so what are you waiting for? Get rid of those extra calories and pounds as early as you can and try to enjoy life the best you can without inviting all those terrible diseases that come with a few extra pounds.

About The Author

Windy Madison is a health junkie. She is very interested in clean eating to have a healthier lifestyle for her family and friends. Through constant research and experimentation, Windy has discovered some amazing tips on clean eating to help attain overall health.

She currently lives and works in New York. In her spare time Windy writes articles about healthy eating on her blog.